Somatic

Exercises for Beginners

"Embark on a Journey to Wellness, Discover Mindful Movement, Transformative Breath, diets, daily routine and Personalized Practices for Holistic Well-Being"

Dr. Fathum

Table of contents

Chapter I. Introduction

A. Understanding Somatic Exercises

Understanding somatic exercises requires delving into the profound philosophy that underlies this transformative practice. Somatics is derived from the Greek word "soma," meaning the living body, and it encompasses a holistic approach to movement and self-awareness. At its core, somatic exercises are not merely physical routines; they are a pathway to unlocking the body's innate intelligence and fostering a deeper connection between mind and body.

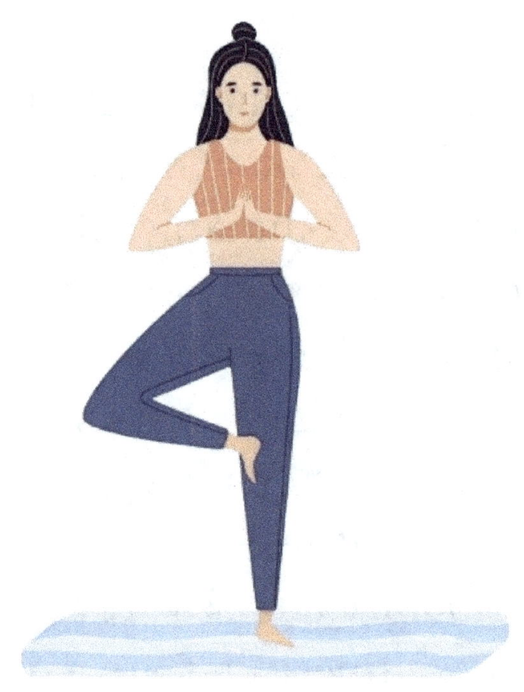

Embodied Wisdom:

Central to the understanding of somatics is the concept of embodied wisdom. Unlike traditional exercise routines that may focus solely on external movements, somatic exercises emphasize turning inward. It's about listening to the body's signals, sensations, and innate intelligence. The body is not seen as a machine to be fixed but as a vessel of wisdom waiting to be explored.

Movement as Inquiry:

In somatics, movement is a form of inquiry. It's not about conforming to external standards but about exploring one's unique range of motion, sensations, and feelings. Through deliberate and mindful movements, individuals engage in a dialogue with their bodies, unraveling layers of tension, and gradually expanding their physical and mental capabilities.

Neuroplasticity and Mind-Body Connection:

Somatic exercises leverage the principles of neuroplasticity, acknowledging the brain's ability to reorganize and adapt. The mind-body connection is a fundamental aspect, recognizing that mental and emotional states influence physical well-being and vice versa. By fostering this connection, somatics empowers individuals to not only improve physical function but also enhance overall mental and emotional resilience.

Release and Relaxation:

Another key aspect of somatic exercises is the emphasis on release and relaxation. Unlike strenuous workouts that may contribute to tension, somatics encourages the release of chronic muscular holding patterns. Through gentle movements and breath awareness, individuals can let go of accumulated stress, promoting a state of deep relaxation that is conducive to healing and restoration.

Cultivating Body Awareness:

A cornerstone of somatic practice is cultivating body awareness. This involves paying attention to the sensations, tensions, and subtle movements within the body. By developing a heightened awareness, individuals can recognize and address imbalances, paving the way for more efficient and effortless movement.

In summary, understanding somatic exercises involves embracing a paradigm shift in how we perceive and engage with our bodies. It's an invitation to move beyond external standards and explore the rich terrain of our internal landscape. Through embodied wisdom, mindful movement, and a deepened mind-body connection, somatics becomes a transformative journey towards greater well-being and self-discovery.

B. Benefits for Beginners

For beginners embarking on the journey of somatic exercises, a myriad of transformative benefits awaits, encompassing physical, mental, and emotional well-being. Here's a comprehensive look at the advantages that make somatic practice particularly rewarding for those just starting:

1. Improved Posture:

Somatic exercises place a strong emphasis on body awareness and alignment. Beginners can experience a gradual improvement in posture as they learn to release tension, align the spine, and move with greater awareness. This not only enhances physical appearance but also contributes to overall musculoskeletal health.

2. Enhanced Flexibility:

Through gentle and mindful movements, beginners engage in a process of dynamic stretching, fostering increased flexibility. Somatic exercises encourage the body to explore its full range of motion, promoting suppleness in muscles and joints. This newfound flexibility contributes to improved mobility and reduces the risk of injuries.

3. Stress Reduction:

Somatic practices integrate breath awareness and relaxation techniques, providing beginners with effective tools to manage stress. As individuals release tension held in the body, they cultivate a sense of calm and relaxation. This, in turn, helps reduce overall stress levels, contributing to better mental and emotional well-being.

4. Heightened Body Awareness:

One of the foundational principles of somatic exercises is cultivating body awareness. Beginners learn to tune into the subtle signals and sensations within their bodies. This heightened awareness allows for a deeper understanding of how emotions and stress manifest physically, empowering individuals to address and release these patterns.

5. Mind-Body Connection:

Somatic exercises emphasize the integral connection between the mind and body. Beginners develop an increased awareness of how thoughts and emotions influence physical sensations. This mind-body connection not only enhances the effectiveness of the exercises but also provides valuable insights into overall well-being.

6. Pain Relief:

For beginners dealing with chronic pain or discomfort, somatic exercises offer a gentle and holistic approach to pain relief. By releasing muscular tension and improving overall body awareness, individuals may find relief from conditions such as back pain, neck tension, and headaches.

7. Improved Sleep Quality:

The relaxation and mindfulness aspects of somatic exercises contribute to improved sleep quality. As individuals release accumulated tension, they create a conducive environment for rest and recovery. Better sleep patterns, in turn, support overall health and vitality.

8. Empowerment and Self-Discovery:

Engaging in somatic exercises is a journey of self-discovery. Beginners often experience a sense of empowerment as they become attuned to their bodies' capabilities and limitations. This self-awareness fosters a positive relationship with one's body, promoting a holistic sense of well-being.

Chapter II. Foundations of Somatics
A. Body Awareness

Body awareness, a foundational principle in somatic exercises, involves cultivating a deep and conscious understanding of one's own body. It goes beyond mere physicality, delving into the intricate relationship between the body, mind, and emotions. Here's a closer look at the significance and components of body awareness in the context of somatic practices:

1. Sensory Perception:

Body awareness begins with tuning into the body's sensory perceptions. It involves paying attention to the sensations, textures, and feelings present within different parts of the body. This heightened sensory awareness enables individuals to discern subtle changes and signals that may indicate areas of tension, discomfort, or relaxation.

2. Movement Awareness:

Understanding how the body moves is a crucial aspect of body awareness in somatic exercises. It entails being mindful of the quality and range of movement, observing how different parts of the body engage in various activities. This awareness fosters a conscious connection with one's physical capabilities and limitations.

3. Breath Awareness:

Somatic practices often incorporate breath awareness as a key component of body awareness. Mindful breathing not only helps individuals stay present in the moment but also provides a gateway to understanding the interplay between breath and bodily sensations. Conscious breathing can be a powerful tool for releasing tension and promoting relaxation.

4. Emotional Awareness:

The body is a repository of emotions, and body awareness extends to recognizing the emotional dimensions housed within. Somatic exercises encourage individuals to explore how emotions manifest physically, whether through tension, knots, or other sensations. This emotional awareness allows for a holistic approach to well-being, addressing both the physical and emotional aspects of one's self.

5. Postural Awareness:

A significant aspect of body awareness is understanding and improving one's posture. Somatic exercises guide individuals in recognizing habitual postural patterns and exploring more optimal alignment. By bringing attention to the spine, pelvis, and overall body structure, individuals can work towards enhancing posture and reducing strain.

6. Mind-Body Connection:

Body awareness in somatic practices is intricately linked to the mind-body connection. It involves acknowledging how thoughts and emotions influence physical sensations and vice versa. This integrated awareness is a key tenet of somatics, emphasizing that the mind and body are not separate entities but interconnected aspects of a unified whole.

7. Release and Relaxation:

As individuals develop body awareness, they gain the ability to consciously release tension held in different parts of the body. This intentional release contributes to a state of relaxation, fostering a sense of ease and fluidity in movement. The process of letting go becomes a powerful tool for promoting overall well-being.

In essence, body awareness in somatic exercises is a journey of self-discovery. It involves becoming attuned to the intricate language of the body, listening to its cues, and fostering a harmonious relationship between the physical, mental, and emotional aspects of one's being. As individuals deepen their body awareness, they unlock the potential for greater self-understanding and holistic well-being.

B. Mind-Body Connection

The mind-body connection is a fundamental concept in somatic exercises, emphasizing the intricate interplay between mental and physical states. It acknowledges that thoughts, emotions, and attitudes profoundly impact the body, and, conversely, the body's condition influences mental and emotional well-being. Understanding and nurturing this connection is pivotal in achieving holistic health and wellness. Here are key aspects of the mind-body connection within the context of somatic practices:

1. Thoughts Influence Physical Sensations:

Somatic exercises recognize that thoughts and mental states manifest physically. Stressful thoughts, for instance, can result in muscle tension, knots, or discomfort. By cultivating awareness, individuals can identify how their mental processes influence their bodies, creating an opportunity for intentional change.

2. Emotions as Embodied Experiences:

Emotions are not isolated to the mind; they are embodied experiences. The mind-body connection in somatic practices involves exploring how emotions are expressed physically. For example, joy may manifest as lightness, while sadness could be accompanied by a sense of heaviness. Acknowledging and expressing these emotions through movement contributes to overall well-being.

3. Breath as a Bridge:

The breath serves as a powerful bridge between the mind and body. Conscious breathing is a central component of somatic exercises, linking mental focus with physical sensations. By directing attention to the breath, individuals can regulate emotions, calm the mind, and influence the body's response to stress.

4. Body Movement Affects Mood:

Somatic practices recognize that intentional body movement can influence mood and mental states. Engaging in mindful and purposeful movements can evoke feelings of relaxation, joy, or empowerment. This bidirectional relationship allows individuals to use movement as a tool for shaping their emotional and mental well-being.

5. Stress Response and Relaxation:

Understanding the mind-body connection involves recognizing the body's stress response and learning techniques to induce relaxation. Somatic exercises guide individuals to release tension, deactivate the stress response, and promote a state of relaxation. This, in turn, positively affects mental clarity and emotional resilience.

6. Body Scan and Mindfulness:

Somatic exercises often include practices like body scans, where individuals systematically direct attention to different parts of their bodies. This mindfulness approach enhances the mind-body connection by fostering awareness of physical sensations, thoughts, and emotions. The result is a more integrated and present experience of the self.

7. Intentional Movement and Neuroplasticity:

The mind-body connection is closely linked to the concept of neuroplasticity, the brain's ability to adapt and reorganize. Intentional and mindful movement in somatic exercises contributes to positive changes in neural pathways, reinforcing a healthier mind-body relationship over time.

By exploring and nurturing the mind-body connection, somatic exercises empower individuals to cultivate a more harmonious and integrated sense of self. This awareness allows for intentional shifts in mental and physical well-being, providing a holistic approach to health that goes beyond the traditional separation of mind and body.

C. Breathing Techniques

In somatic exercises, breathing techniques play a pivotal role in fostering a mindful connection between the body and mind. These techniques go beyond simple inhalation and exhalation, serving as a powerful tool to promote relaxation, enhance body awareness, and synchronize breath with intentional movements. Here are some key breathing techniques commonly used in somatic practices:

1. Diaphragmatic Breathing:

Also known as belly breathing, diaphragmatic breathing involves drawing the breath deep into the lungs, allowing the diaphragm to descend. This technique is foundational in somatic exercises, promoting relaxation and reducing the activation of the body's stress response. It also enhances oxygenation and supports a calm and centered state.

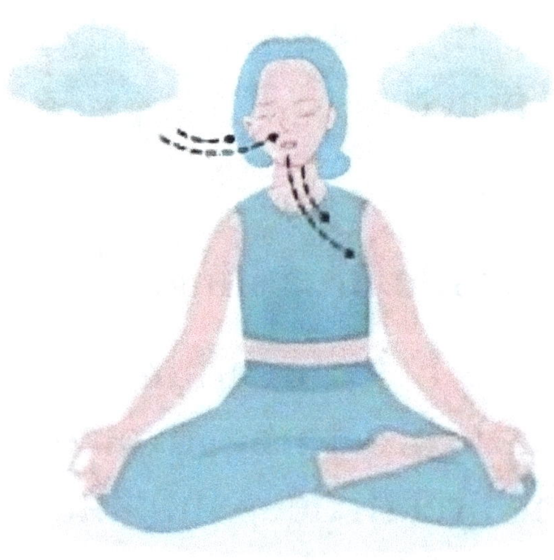

2. Rib-Cage Breathing:

Rib-cage breathing focuses on expanding the ribcage laterally while breathing in and allowing it to contract during exhalation. This technique helps improve the mobility of the ribcage and promotes a fuller, more expansive breath. Rib-cage breathing is often integrated into somatic exercises to enhance overall lung capacity.

3. Three-Part Breath:

The three-part breath involves sequentially filling three areas of the lungs – the lower, middle, and upper regions. This technique encourages a complete and deep breath, fostering a sense of full-body expansion. It is particularly effective in promoting relaxation and increasing body awareness.

4. Coordinated Breath and Movement:

In somatic exercises, coordinating breath with specific movements is key to enhancing the mind-body connection. Whether it's inhaling during a gentle stretch or exhaling during a release, synchronizing breath and movement fosters a sense of unity and mindfulness. This intentional coordination encourages a fluid and integrated experience.

5. Equal-Length Breathing:

Equal-length breathing involves inhaling and exhaling for the same duration, creating a balanced and rhythmic breath pattern. This technique promotes a sense of calm and can be used as a grounding practice in somatic exercises, helping individuals stay present and centered.

6. Guided Breath Meditation:

Somatic exercises often incorporate guided breath meditations, where individuals are led through intentional breathing patterns. These guided sessions can range from focusing on the sensations of breath to visualizing the breath moving through different parts of the body. Guided breath meditations contribute to relaxation and heightened body awareness.

7. Breath Awareness in Resting Positions:

Even in stillness, somatic practices emphasize maintaining awareness of the breath. Whether lying down or sitting in a relaxed position, individuals are encouraged to observe the natural rhythm of their breath. This breath awareness fosters a meditative state and supports the overall calming effects of somatic exercises.

8. Mindful Exhalation for Relaxation:

Conscious emphasis on the exhale is a common technique in somatic practices. Lengthening the exhalation engages the body's relaxation response, encouraging the release of tension. Mindful exhalation is particularly effective in promoting a sense of ease and calmness.

Incorporating these breathing techniques into somatic exercises allows individuals to tap into the profound connection between breath and movement. As a result, practitioners can experience not only physical benefits such as improved oxygenation but also enhanced mental clarity, reduced stress, and a deeper sense of presence in their somatic journey.

Chapter III. Getting Started

A. Preparing Your Space

Creating a conducive and mindful space is crucial when engaging in somatic exercises. The environment in which you practice can significantly impact your ability to focus, relax, and connect with your body. Here are key considerations for preparing your space for somatic exercises:

1. Quiet and Distraction-Free:

Choose a quiet and distraction-free space for your somatic practice. Turn off electronic devices and minimize external noise to create an environment that allows you to fully immerse yourself in the exercises. This sets the stage for a more mindful and focused experience.

2. Comfortable Flooring:

Opt for a comfortable and supportive surface, such as a yoga mat or carpet, for your somatic exercises. This ensures a pleasant experience during floor-based movements and provides a cushioning effect for joints. If you're practicing seated or standing exercises, make sure the surface is stable and non-slip.

3. Adequate Lighting:

Ensure that the lighting in your space is sufficient for your somatic practice. Natural light is ideal, but if that's not possible, use soft and ambient artificial lighting. A well-lit space enhances your ability to maintain awareness of your body and movements.

4. Temperature Control:

Maintain a comfortable temperature in your practice space. Ensure proper ventilation and consider the climate to avoid discomfort during exercises. Dress in layers, so you can adjust accordingly as your body temperature changes during the practice.

5. Clear Space:

Clear the area of any obstacles or clutter. Having ample space around you allows for unrestricted movement, reducing the risk of accidental bumps or trips. A clutter-free space contributes to a sense of openness and promotes a more mindful practice.

6. Supportive Props:

Depending on the somatic exercises you plan to engage in, consider using supportive props like yoga blocks, cushions, or a blanket. These props can enhance your comfort and provide additional support during certain movements or relaxation postures.

7. Mindful Décor:

Infuse your space with elements that promote mindfulness and relaxation. Consider incorporating soothing colors, plants, or objects that hold personal significance. Creating an environment that aligns with your intention for the somatic practice contributes to a more holistic experience.

8. Personalized Ambiance:

Tailor the ambiance of your space to your preferences. Whether it's playing calming music, using aromatherapy, or having a scented candle, these elements can enhance the sensory experience of your somatic exercises and contribute to a more serene atmosphere.

9. Uninterrupted Time:

Allocate uninterrupted time for your somatic practice. Inform household members or colleagues about your designated practice time to minimize disruptions. This ensures that you can fully engage in the exercises without external distractions.

By thoughtfully preparing your space, you create a supportive and harmonious environment for your somatic journey. A well-prepared space enhances your ability to connect with your body, fosters mindfulness, and contributes to a more fulfilling and beneficial somatic practice.

B. Warm-up Exercises

A proper warm-up is essential before engaging in somatic exercises, preparing the body for mindful movement and promoting flexibility. Here are some gentle and effective warm-up exercises suitable for a somatic practice:

1. Breath Awareness:

Begin with a few minutes of focused breath awareness. In a comfortable seated or standing position, take slow and deep breaths, bringing attention to the inhale and exhale. This calms the nervous system and centers your focus on the present moment.

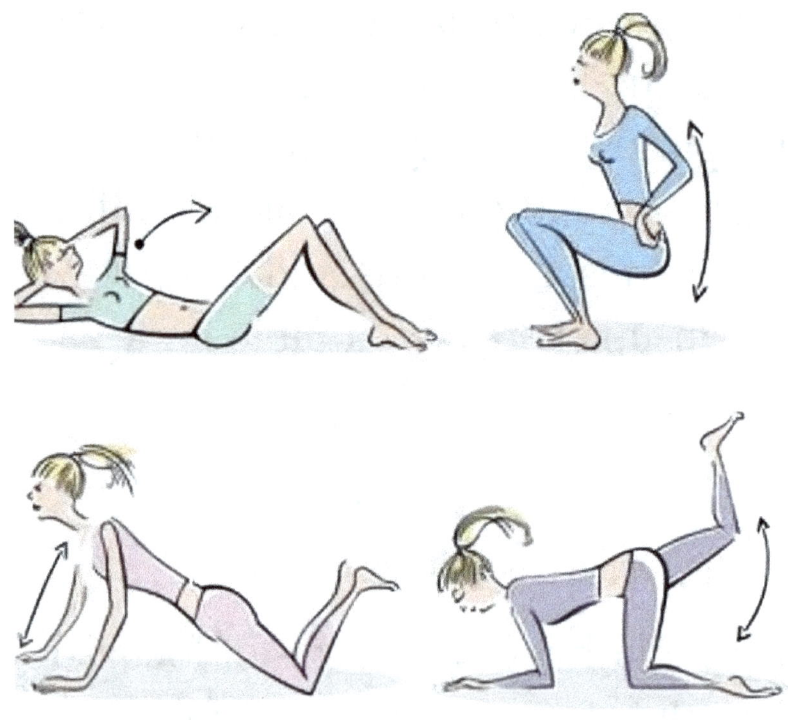

2. Neck and Shoulder Rolls:

Slowly and mindfully roll your shoulders in a circular motion, both clockwise and counterclockwise. Follow this with gentle neck rolls, moving your head in a circular motion, allowing the neck muscles to release tension. Ensure movements are slow and controlled.

3. Spinal Warm-up:

Sit or stand with a straight spine. Inhale, lengthening your spine, and as you exhale, gently twist your torso to one side. Inhale back to the center and exhale to the other side. Repeat this movement several times, encouraging a gradual release in the spine.

4. Side Stretches:

While standing or sitting, extend one arm overhead and gently lean to the opposite side, creating a lateral stretch along the torso. Hold for a few breaths, then switch sides. This movement promotes flexibility in the side body.

5. Gentle Forward Fold:

Stand with feet hip-width apart. Inhale to lengthen the spine, and as you exhale, hinge at the hips and let your upper body fold forward. Keep the knees slightly bent. This gentle forward fold helps release tension in the lower back and hamstrings.

6. Hip Circles:

Stand with feet hip-width apart. Circle your hips in a gentle, fluid motion, first clockwise and then counterclockwise. This movement warms up the hip joints and promotes mobility.

7. Ankle and Wrist Rolls:

Sit comfortably and roll your ankles in both directions. Follow this with gentle wrist rolls. These simple movements help warm up the joints in your extremities, preparing them for more dynamic somatic exercises.

8. Mindful Walking:

Take a few minutes for mindful walking. Focus on each step, feeling the connection between your feet and the ground. This prepares the body for weight-bearing movements and promotes awareness of your body's relationship with space.

9. Full-Body Shaking:

Stand with feet hip-width apart and shake your body gently. Allow the arms, legs, and torso to shake freely. This dynamic movement helps release tension, increases blood flow, and prepares the body for more intentional somatic exercises.

Remember to perform these warm-up exercises slowly and mindfully, paying attention to your breath and sensations. The goal is to increase blood flow, enhance flexibility, and bring a heightened awareness to your body before diving into more specific somatic movements.

Chapter IV. Core Somatic Exercises

A. Neck and Shoulder Release

For a targeted neck and shoulder release in somatic exercises, consider the following gentle and mindful movements. These exercises can help alleviate tension and promote relaxation in these areas:

1. Neck Stretch:

- Sit or stand comfortably with a straight spine.

- Slowly tilt your head to one side, bringing your ear towards your shoulder.

- Hold the stretch for a few breaths,
feeling a gentle stretch along the side

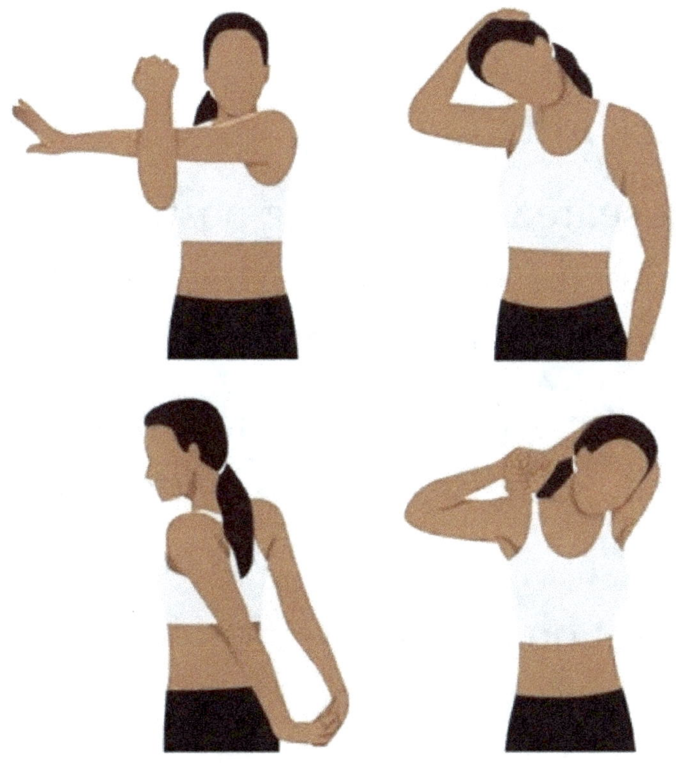

of your neck.

- Repeat on the other side.

- Avoid forcing the stretch; keep it gentle and within a comfortable range of motion.

2. Neck Rotation:

- In a seated or standing position, turn your head to one side, bringing your chin towards your shoulder.

- Hold for a few breaths, feeling a stretch along the opposite side of your neck.

- Repeat on the other side.

- Move slowly and with awareness, allowing the neck muscles to release tension.

3. Shoulder Rolls:

- While seated or standing, roll your shoulders in a circular motion.

- Inhale as you lift your shoulders towards your ears, and exhale as you roll them back and down.

- Repeat this movement for several rounds, allowing the shoulders to relax and release tension.

4. Shoulder Stretch:

- Bring your right arm across your chest.

- Use your left hand to gently press the right arm closer to your chest, feeling a stretch in the outer part of the shoulder.

- Hold for a few breaths, then switch sides.

- Maintain a relaxed breath throughout the stretch.

5. Neck Self-Massage:

- Use your fingertips to gently massage the base of your skull, moving in circular motions.

- Gradually work your way down the neck, applying gentle pressure where you feel tension.

- This self-massage helps release knots and tightness in the neck muscles.

6. Shoulder Blade Squeeze:

- Sit or stand with a straight spine.

- Inhale as you squeeze your shoulder blades together, opening your chest.

- Exhale as you release the squeeze.

- Repeat this movement several times to promote mobility and release tension in the upper back.

7. Ear-to-Shoulder Stretch:

- Slowly lower one ear towards the corresponding shoulder, feeling a gentle stretch along the side of your neck.

- Hold for a few breaths, then switch to the other side.

- Keep the movements slow and controlled, avoiding any sudden or forceful stretches.

8. Mindful Breathing:

- Incorporate mindful breathing throughout these exercises. Inhale deeply through the nose, and exhale slowly through the mouth.

- Use your breath to enhance relaxation and release tension in the neck and shoulders.

Perform these neck and shoulder release exercises with awareness, focusing on the sensations and allowing the muscles to gradually release tension. If you experience any pain or discomfort, adjust the movements to better suit your comfort level. These gentle exercises can be incorporated into your somatic routine to promote flexibility and ease in the neck and shoulder area.

B. Spinal Alignment Techniques

Maintaining proper spinal alignment is fundamental for overall well-being, and somatic exercises offer effective techniques to support a healthy spine.

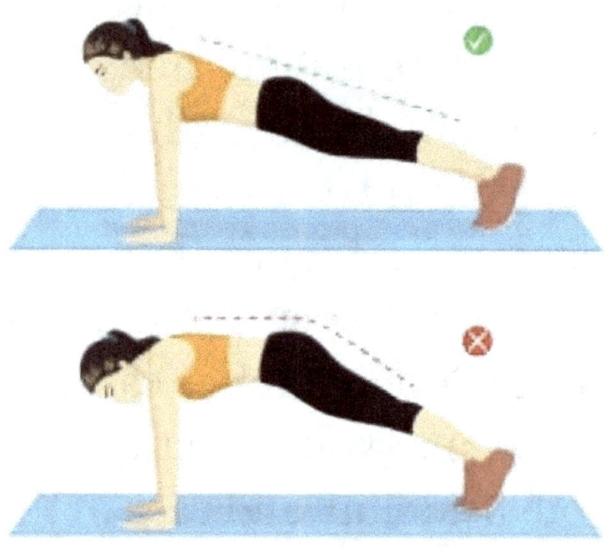

Here are gentle and mindful spinal alignment techniques to promote flexibility and alleviate tension:

1. Seated Spinal Twist:

- Sit comfortably with a straight spine.

- Inhale, lengthening your spine, and as you exhale, twist your torso to one side.

- Place one hand on the opposite knee and the other hand behind you for support.

- Hold the twist for a few breaths, feeling the gentle rotation along the spine.

- Inhale back to the center and repeat on the other side.

2. Cat-Cow Stretch:

- Start on your hands and knees in a tabletop position.

- Inhale as you arch your back, dropping your belly towards the floor (Cow Pose).

- Exhale as you round your spine, tucking your chin to your chest (Cat Pose).

- Flow between these two positions, coordinating the movement with your breath.

- This dynamic stretch promotes flexibility and mobility along the entire spine.

3. Forward Fold:

- Stand with your feet hip-width apart.

- Inhale as you lengthen your spine, and as you exhale, hinge at the hips and fold forward.

- Allow your upper body to hang, and let your head and neck relax.

- Bend your knees slightly if needed, focusing on releasing tension along the spine.

4. Child's Pose:

- Start in a kneeling position with your toes touching and knees apart.

- Sit back on your heels and extend your arms forward, lowering your chest towards the floor.

- Rest your forehead on the ground and let your spine lengthen in this gentle stretch.

- Breathe deeply into the back of your ribcage.

5. Bridge Pose:

- Lie on your back with your knees bent and feet hip-width apart.

- Inhale as you lift your hips towards the ceiling, pressing into your feet.

- Keep your shoulders grounded and engage your core.

- Hold the bridge position for a few breaths, feeling the lengthening of the spine.

6. Somatic Pelvic Tilt:

- Lie on your back with knees bent and feet hip-width apart.

- Inhale to prepare, and as you exhale, tilt your pelvis towards you, creating a small arch in your lower back.

- Inhale to return to the neutral position.

- Repeat this pelvic tilting movement, focusing on the gentle articulation of the spine.

7. Standing Side Bend:

- Stand with feet hip-width apart.

- Inhale as you reach one arm overhead, lengthening the spine.

- Exhale and bend to the side, creating a gentle stretch along the length of your spine.

- Inhale back to the center and repeat on the other side.

8. Gentle Spinal Rotation:

- Sit comfortably with a straight spine.

- Inhale and lengthen your spine, and as you exhale, rotate your torso to one side.

- Place one hand behind you for support and the other on your outer knee.

- Hold the rotation for a few breaths, feeling the twist along your spine.

- Inhale back to the center and repeat on the other side.

Practice these spinal alignment techniques mindfully, paying attention to the sensations and allowing the movements to flow with your breath. Incorporating these exercises into your somatic routine can contribute to a more flexible, aligned, and healthy spine over time.

C.   Pelvic Floor Activation

Activating and strengthening the pelvic floor is an integral aspect of somatic exercises, contributing to overall core stability, posture, and even pelvic health. Here are mindful pelvic floor activation techniques to incorporate into your somatic practice:

1. Pelvic Tilts:

- Lie on your back with knees bent and feet hip-width apart.

- Inhale, engaging your core, and as you exhale, tilt your pelvis towards you, creating a small arch in your lower back.

- Inhale to return to the neutral position.

- Exhale and tilt your pelvis away from you, gently pressing your lower back into the floor.

- Repeat this pelvic tilting movement, focusing on the controlled engagement of the pelvic floor muscles.

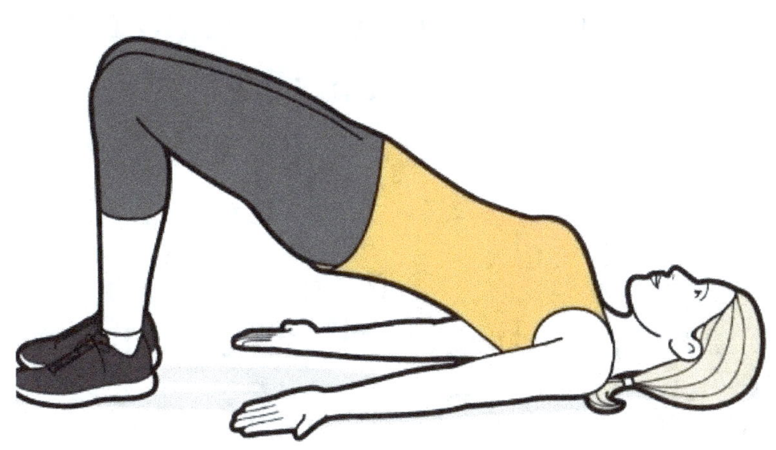

2. Kegel Exercises:

- Sit or lie comfortably.

- Identify your pelvic floor muscles by imagining stopping the flow of urine midstream.

- Once identified, contract these muscles, lifting and squeezing them.

- Hold the contraction for a few seconds, then release.

- Repeat these contractions in sets, gradually increasing the duration of the holds as your strength improves.

3. Pelvic Clock:

- Lie on your back with knees bent and feet hip-width apart.

- Imagine your pelvis as the center of a clock.

- Begin tilting your pelvis to 12 o'clock (towards your head), then move to 6 o'clock (away from your head).

- Continue this movement to 3 o'clock and 9 o'clock.

- Explore all points on the "clock" to engage and activate different aspects of the pelvic floor.

4. Bridge Pose with Pelvic Floor Engagement:

- Lie on your back with knees bent and feet hip-width apart.

- Inhale as you lift your hips towards the ceiling, engaging your glutes.

- As you lift, also engage your pelvic floor muscles by imagining a gentle lift and squeeze.

- Hold the bridge position for a few breaths, focusing on the activation of the pelvic floor.

5. Seated Pelvic Floor Activation:

- Sit comfortably with a straight spine.

- Inhale deeply, engaging your core, and as you exhale, lift and squeeze your pelvic floor muscles.

- Hold the contraction for a few seconds, then release.

- Repeat this seated activation, connecting the breath with the engagement of the pelvic floor.

6. Squatting with Pelvic Floor Engagement:

- Stand with feet hip-width apart.

- Inhale as you lower into a squat position, keeping your knees aligned with your feet.

- As you exhale, engage your pelvic floor muscles, lifting and squeezing.

- Inhale to rise back to the standing position.

- Repeat the squatting movement, integrating pelvic floor activation.

7. Supine Butterfly Stretch:

- Lie on your back with knees bent and soles of your feet together, allowing your knees to fall outward.

- Inhale deeply, and as you exhale, engage your pelvic floor muscles, gently pressing your lower back into the floor.

- Hold the stretch for a few breaths, feeling the engagement in the pelvic floor.

8. Standing Pelvic Floor Activation:

- Stand with feet hip-width apart.

- Inhale deeply, and as you exhale, lift and squeeze your pelvic floor muscles.

- Hold the contraction for a few seconds, then release.

- Repeat this standing activation, maintaining good posture and connecting the breath with pelvic floor engagement.

Practice these pelvic floor activation techniques with mindfulness and control. Over time, incorporating these exercises into your somatic routine can contribute to improved pelvic floor strength, stability, and overall well-being. If you have any concerns or specific health conditions, it's advisable to consult with a healthcare professional or a qualified somatic instructor.

Chapter V. Mindful Movement Sequences

A.   Integration of Breath and Movement

The integration of breath and movement is a foundational principle in somatic exercises, fostering a harmonious connection between the body and breath. This synchronization enhances mindfulness, body awareness, and the overall effectiveness of the somatic practice. Here are ways to integrate breath and movement seamlessly:

1. Mindful Breath Initiation:

- Begin each movement with a mindful inhalation or exhalation.

- Inhale to prepare the body for the upcoming movement, and exhale as you initiate the motion.

- This conscious breath initiation sets the tone for a focused and connected somatic experience.

2. Coordinated Flow:

- Coordinate each movement with the natural rhythm of your breath.

- For example, in a gentle stretch, inhale as you lengthen, and exhale as you release or deepen the stretch.

- Maintain a fluid and intentional connection between your breath and the flow of movements.

3. Full-Bodied Breathing:

- Emphasize full-bodied breathing, allowing the breath to expand into the entire lung capacity.

- During dynamic movements, encourage deep inhalations and complete exhalations to support the engagement of the diaphragm and enhance oxygenation.

4. Breath Awareness During Holds:

- When holding a posture or stretch, maintain awareness of your breath.

- Avoid holding the breath and instead focus on maintaining a steady and mindful rhythm.

- Use the breath to explore any areas of tension or resistance within the posture.

5. Breath as a Guide for Range of Motion:

- Allow your breath to guide the range of motion in each movement.

- Inhale to explore expansion and lengthening, and exhale to release and soften.

- This approach promotes a dynamic and responsive interaction between your breath and body.

6. Breath-Centric Meditation:

- Integrate breath-centric meditation into your somatic practice.

- Take moments of stillness to focus solely on your breath, bringing awareness to the sensations of inhalation and exhalation.

- This mindfulness practice enhances the mind-body connection.

7. Breath Pacing in Dynamic Movements:

- When engaging in dynamic movements, synchronize the pace of your breath with the pace of the movement.

- For instance, in a sequence of flowing stretches, match the inhalations and exhalations to the rhythm of the movements for a seamless integration.

8. Breath-Cued Transitions:

- Use your breath as a cue for smooth transitions between movements.

- Inhale to transition into a new posture or movement, and exhale as you settle into the position.

- This breath-aware approach enhances the fluidity of the somatic sequence.

By consciously integrating breath and movement, somatic exercises become a holistic practice that goes beyond physical flexibility and strength. This mindful connection fosters a deeper sense of awareness, relaxation, and presence throughout the entire somatic experience. As you explore the integration of breath and movement, allow it to become a natural and intuitive part of your somatic routine.

B. Exploring Range of Motion

Exploring range of motion in somatic exercises is a key component to enhance flexibility, joint mobility, and overall body awareness. Here's a brief guide on how to effectively explore and improve your range of motion:

1. Mindful Warm-up:

   - Begin with a mindful warm-up to prepare your body for movement.

   - Incorporate gentle joint rotations and dynamic stretches to increase blood flow and flexibility.

2. Joint-Specific Movements:

- Focus on specific joints, such as shoulders, hips, knees, and ankles.

- Perform controlled and intentional movements to explore the full range of motion in each joint.

3. Dynamic Stretches:

- Engage in dynamic stretches that involve continuous, fluid movements.

- Gradually increase the intensity and range of your stretches, respecting your body's comfort levels.

4. Somatic Exercises:

- Integrate somatic exercises that encourage mindful exploration of your body's capabilities.

- Emphasize movements that engage multiple joints, promoting overall flexibility and coordination.

5. Breath Awareness:

- Coordinate your breath with your movements.

- Inhale to expand and create space, exhale to release tension and explore deeper into your range of motion.

6. Progressive Approach:

- Progress gradually, especially if you're working on increasing flexibility.

- Avoid forcing movements and instead focus on gentle, progressive stretches.

7. Targeted Stretching:

- Identify areas of your body that may have restricted mobility.

- Incorporate targeted stretching exercises to address specific muscle groups and joints.

8. Prop Assistance:

- Utilize props like yoga blocks or straps to assist in achieving a greater range of motion.

- Props can provide support and enable you to explore stretches more comfortably.

9. Mind-Body Connection:

- Cultivate a strong mind-body connection during your explorations.

- Tune into the sensations within your body, distinguishing between discomfort and pain.

10. Regular Practice:

   - Consistency is key to seeing improvements in your range of motion.

   - Include range of motion exercises as a regular part of your somatic practice.

11. Post-Exploration Reflection:

   - Take a moment after each session to reflect on your experience.

   - Note any changes in your range of motion, areas of improvement, or insights gained during the exploration.

Remember to approach the exploration of range of motion with patience, mindfulness, and a deep respect for your body's unique capabilities. Regular practice and a gradual progression will contribute to increased flexibility and a heightened awareness of your body's movement potential.

Chapter VI. Progressive Relaxation Techniques

A. Guided Muscle Relaxation

Guided muscle relaxation is a powerful technique to release tension, promote relaxation, and enhance overall well-being. Here's a step-by-step guide to help you practice guided muscle relaxation:

1. Find a Comfortable Position:

   - Sit or lie down in a comfortable position. Ensure your body is supported, and you won't be disturbed during the practice.

2. Close Your Eyes:

   - Gently close your eyes to minimize external distractions and turn your focus inward.

3. Deep Breathing:

   - Begin with a few deep breaths to center yourself.

   - Inhale slowly through your nose, allowing your abdomen to expand. Exhale slowly through your mouth, releasing any tension with each breath.

4. Body Scan:

- Bring your attention to different parts of your body, starting from your toes and moving upward.

- As you focus on each body part, consciously release any tension or tightness you may be holding.

5. Progressive Muscle Relaxation:

- Start with your toes, intentionally tensing the muscles for a few seconds, then release and let the tension melt away.

- Move to your feet, calves, thighs, and progressively work your way up through each muscle group, including your abdomen, chest, arms, neck, and face.

6. Visualize Warmth and Relaxation:

   - As you release tension, visualize a warm, soothing sensation spreading through each relaxed muscle.

   - Imagine this warmth promoting deep relaxation and a sense of tranquility.

7. Affirmations:

   - Include positive affirmations related to relaxation and well-being.

   - For example, silently repeat phrases like "I am calm and at ease" or "My body is relaxed, and my mind is peaceful."

8. Breath Awareness Throughout:

   - Maintain awareness of your breath throughout the process.

   - Allow your breath to remain steady and calming, syncing it with the release of tension in each muscle group.

9. Hold and Release:

   - Hold the tension in each muscle group for a few seconds before releasing.

   - Focus on the contrast between tension and relaxation.

10. Complete Body Relaxation:

- Once you've scanned and released tension in each part of your body, experience the overall sensation of relaxation.

- Enjoy a few moments of complete muscle relaxation, allowing yourself to rest in this state.

11. Transition Slowly:

- When you're ready to conclude the practice, transition slowly.

- Gently wiggle your fingers and toes, gradually bringing awareness back to your surroundings.

12. Open Your Eyes:

- When you feel ready, open your eyes, and take a moment to reorient yourself to the present moment.

Guided muscle relaxation can be a rejuvenating practice, promoting physical and mental relaxation. Incorporate this technique into your routine, especially during times of stress or before bedtime, to experience its calming benefits.

B. Stress Release through Somatics

Stress release through somatics involves utilizing mindful movement, breath awareness, and the mind-body connection to alleviate tension and promote a sense of calm. Here's a guide on how to release stress through somatic practices:

1. Mindful Body Awareness:

  - Begin by bringing attention to your body.

  - Notice areas of tension or discomfort without judgment, simply observing sensations.

2. Gentle Breathing Techniques:

  - Practice slow, deep breaths to initiate relaxation.

- Inhale deeply through your nose, allowing your abdomen to expand. Exhale slowly through your mouth, releasing tension with each breath.

3. Somatic Exercises:

   - Engage in gentle somatic movements to release physical tension.

   - Focus on movements that encourage a fluid and mindful exploration of your body.

4. Neck and Shoulder Release:

   - Perform slow and deliberate movements to release tension in the neck and shoulders.

- Incorporate gentle stretches and rotations to promote relaxation.

5. Spinal Alignment Techniques:

- Pay attention to your spine, a common area where stress is stored.

- Practice somatic exercises that promote alignment and flexibility in the spine.

6. Pelvic Floor Activation and Release:

- Explore somatic exercises targeting the pelvic area.

- Activate and release the pelvic floor muscles to release tension and promote relaxation.

7. Integration of Breath and Movement:

   - Coordinate breath with movement to deepen the mind-body connection.

   - Inhale during the preparatory phase, and exhale as you release tension during the movement.

8. Mindful Transitions:

   - Emphasize smooth transitions between different somatic exercises.

   - Allow each movement to flow seamlessly into the next, promoting a sense of continuity and ease.

9. Creative Movement Exploration:

   - Incorporate spontaneous, free-form movements.

   - Allow your body to guide you in creative and intuitive movements, expressing and releasing stress.

10. Fine-tuning Mind-Body Harmony:

   - Focus on fine-tuning your mind-body connection during each somatic practice.

   - Cultivate a heightened awareness of sensations, movements, and breath.

11. Somatic Meditation Practices:

- Include moments of stillness and meditation within your somatic routine.

- Practice mindfulness meditation to further release mental and emotional stress.

12. Reflective Journaling:

- Journal about your experience after each session.

- Note any changes in your stress levels, areas of tension release, or insights gained during the practice.

Stress release through somatics is an ongoing process. By incorporating these practices into your routine, you can cultivate a deeper sense of relaxation, resilience, and well-being. Regular engagement with somatic stress release techniques can contribute to a more balanced and harmonious state of being.

Chapter VII. Somatics for Daily Life

A. Incorporating Exercises into Routine

Incorporating somatic exercises into your routine can enhance your overall well-being and contribute to a mindful lifestyle. Here's a guide on seamlessly integrating these exercises into your daily schedule:

1. Establish a Consistent Time:

   - Choose a consistent time each day to practice somatic exercises. This could be in the morning to energize your day or in the evening to unwind.

2. Create a Dedicated Space:

- Designate a quiet and comfortable space for your somatic practice. Having a specific area helps signal the transition into a mindful practice.

3. Start with Short Sessions:

- Begin with shorter sessions, especially if you're new to somatic exercises. A 10-15 minute routine can be effective and easier to integrate into your daily schedule.

4. Morning Wake-Up Routine:

- Incorporate somatic exercises as part of your morning routine to awaken your body and mind. Focus on gentle movements and breath awareness to kickstart your day.

5. Lunchtime Refresh:

- Use your lunch break to engage in a quick somatic session. It can help relieve midday tension and reenergize you for the remainder of the day.

6. Afternoon Pick-Me-Up:

- Combat afternoon fatigue by incorporating somatic exercises. Choose movements that increase circulation and improve focus.

7. Evening Relaxation Ritual:

   - Wind down in the evening with a longer somatic practice. Emphasize relaxation techniques and gentle stretches to prepare your body for rest.

8. Combine with Other Activities:

   - Integrate somatic exercises into existing routines. For example, while waiting for your coffee to brew or during a short break at work, engage in a few mindful movements.

9. Mindful Commuting:

- If you commute, consider incorporating seated somatic exercises or mindful breathing during your journey to promote relaxation.

10. Weekend Exploration:

- Dedicate a bit more time on weekends to explore new somatic exercises or engage in a more extended practice session.

11. Involve Family or Friends:

- Encourage family or friends to join your somatic sessions. It can become a shared activity and promote a supportive environment.

12. Reflect and Adjust:

   - Regularly reflect on your somatic practice. Adjust the duration and intensity based on your energy levels and schedule.

13. Use Technology Wisely:

   - Utilize apps or online resources that offer guided somatic exercises. This can be helpful, especially if you prefer structured guidance.

14. Set Reminders:

   - Set daily reminders on your phone or calendar to prompt your somatic practice. Consistent reminders can help establish a routine.

Remember that the key to successful integration is consistency and adaptability. Start small, be mindful of your body's needs, and gradually expand your somatic routine as it becomes a natural part of your daily life.

B. Enhancing Posture and Ergonomics

Improving posture and optimizing ergonomics are crucial for overall well-being, and somatic exercises offer effective techniques to enhance these aspects. Here are mindful practices to promote better posture and ergonomics:

1. Somatic Posture Exploration:

- Begin with a somatic exploration of your current posture.

- Sit or stand comfortably and bring awareness to how you hold your body.

- Notice any areas of tension, imbalance, or habitual postural patterns without judgment.

2. Breath and Posture Alignment:

- Incorporate breath awareness to enhance posture.

- Inhale deeply, lengthening your spine, and exhale, releasing any unnecessary tension.

- Use your breath to maintain an upright and aligned posture throughout daily activities.

3. Core Engagement for Stability:

- Engage your core muscles mindfully to provide stability and support for your spine.

- Somatic exercises that focus on gentle core activation can contribute to improved posture.

4. Dynamic Sitting and Standing:

- Avoid prolonged static positions.

- Incorporate dynamic sitting and standing throughout the day. Change positions regularly to prevent stiffness and enhance blood circulation.

5. Somatic Movement Breaks:

- Take short somatic movement breaks during work or other sedentary activities.

- Perform gentle stretches, rotations, or movements to release tension and re-establish better posture.

6. Mindful Walking and Alignment:

- Practice mindful walking to improve overall posture and gait.

- Pay attention to how your feet connect with the ground and how your spine aligns with each step.

- Let the movement be coordinated with your breath.

7. Ergonomic Workspace Adjustments:

- Assess and adjust your workspace ergonomics.

- Ensure that your chair, desk, and computer are set up to support a neutral spine and comfortable posture.

- Use props or cushions to maintain proper alignment.

8. Body Scan for Tension Release:

- Perform regular body scans to identify and release tension.

- Starting from your head, systematically move through different body parts, releasing tension and promoting relaxation.

- This practice contributes to an overall sense of ease in your posture.

9. Mindful Standing Posture:

- When standing, distribute your weight evenly between both feet.

- Engage your abdominal muscles
gently and avoid locking your knees.

- Align your head, shoulders, and hips
in a straight line for optimal standing
posture.

10. Somatic Exercises for Spinal Mobility:

- Include somatic exercises that
specifically address spinal mobility.

- Movements like gentle twists, side
bends, and stretches can enhance the
flexibility and alignment of the spine.

11. Somatic Shoulder and Neck Releases:

- Address shoulder and neck tension through somatic exercises.

- Perform gentle shoulder rolls, neck stretches, and releases to alleviate stiffness and improve upper body posture.

12. Mindful Body Awareness:

- Cultivate overall body awareness.

- Regularly check in with your body, observing how it feels and adjusting your posture accordingly.

- Develop a mindful approach to movements and daily activities.

Consistent integration of these somatic practices into your routine can contribute to improved posture, reduced tension, and enhanced ergonomics. As you bring mindfulness to your daily movements and activities, you'll foster a more aligned and comfortable relationship with your body.

C. Daily routine

30-Day Daily Routine for Somatic Exercises for Beginners

Weeks 1-2: Foundation Building

Days 1-7: Introduction and Body Awareness

1. Day 1: Welcome Session

   - Introduction to somatic exercises.

   - Body awareness meditation.

2. Day 2-4: Gentle Body Scans

   - Focus on different body regions each day.

   - Notice tension and release through breath awareness.

3. Day 5-7: Mindful Breathing

   - Explore diaphragmatic breathing.

- Connect breath with simple movements.

Days 8-14: Core Concepts and Warm-up Routines

4. Day 8-10: Core Engagement

   - Introduce gentle core activation exercises.

   - Emphasize stability in movement.

5. Day 11-14: Warm-up Flow

   - Develop a 10-minute warm-up routine.

- Include neck, shoulders, and spine movements.

Weeks 3-4: Building Flexibility and Coordination

Days 15-21: Progressive Movements

6. Day 15-18: Joint Mobility

   - Focus on gentle joint movements.

   - Enhance flexibility in wrists, ankles, and hips.

7. Day 19-21: Dynamic Stretches

   - Introduce dynamic stretches.

- Coordinate breath with fluid movements.

8. Day 22-25: Seated Postures

  - Explore seated somatic postures.

  - Emphasize spine alignment and breath integration.

Days 26-30: Integration and Mindfulness

9. Day 26-28: Flowing Sequences

  - Combine learned movements into flowing sequences.

  - Emphasize smooth transitions.

10. Day 29-30: Mindful Integration

   - Practice somatic exercises with closed eyes.

   - Focus on deepening mind-body connection.

Tips for a Successful 30-Day Journey:

- Consistency is Key: Aim for daily practice but be forgiving if you miss a day.

- Listen to Your Body: Modify exercises as needed, and avoid pushing beyond comfort.

- Journaling: Keep a daily journal to track progress, sensations, and insights.

- Celebrate Milestones: Acknowledge achievements and improvements along the way.

By following this 30-day routine, beginners can gradually build a foundation in somatic exercises, fostering mindfulness, flexibility, and a deeper connection with their bodies.

D. Suggested diets

Suggested Diets for Somatic Exercises for Beginners

Proper nutrition plays a crucial role in supporting your body's ability to engage in somatic exercises effectively. Here are some dietary suggestions for beginners incorporating somatic practices into their wellness journey:

1. Hydration:

   - Start your day with a glass of water to rehydrate your body after sleep.

   - Drink water consistently throughout the day to maintain optimal hydration levels.

2. Balanced Meals:

- Prioritize balanced meals that include a mix of lean proteins, whole grains, fruits, and vegetables.

- Aim for a variety of colors on your plate to ensure a diverse range of nutrients.

3. Whole Foods:

- Choose whole, minimally processed foods over highly processed options.

- Incorporate whole grains, fresh fruits, vegetables, and lean proteins into your meals.

4. Anti-Inflammatory Foods:

- Include foods rich in anti-inflammatory properties, such as fatty fish (salmon, mackerel), nuts, seeds, and colorful vegetables.

- Reduce processed foods and those high in added sugars, which can contribute to inflammation.

5. Protein for Muscle Support:

- Ensure an adequate intake of protein to support muscle health and recovery.

- Sources include lean meats, poultry, fish, legumes, and plant-based proteins.

6. Healthy Fats:

   - Incorporate healthy fats from sources like avocados, nuts, seeds, and olive oil.

   - These fats support overall health, including joint flexibility and cognitive function.

7. Pre-Exercise Nutrition:

   - Consume a light, balanced meal or snack 1-2 hours before your somatic exercise session.

   - This might include a combination of carbohydrates and protein for sustained energy.

8. Post-Exercise Nutrition:

   - After your somatic practice, prioritize a meal or snack that includes protein for muscle recovery and carbohydrates for replenishing energy stores.

   - Options might include a protein smoothie, yogurt with fruit, or a balanced meal.

9. Mindful Eating:

   - Practice mindful eating to cultivate awareness around hunger and fullness cues.

   - Avoid distractions while eating and savor each bite.

10. Adequate Vitamin and Mineral
Intake:

- Ensure you're meeting your daily
requirements for essential vitamins
and minerals through a varied and
nutrient-rich diet.

- Consider consulting with a
healthcare professional for
personalized guidance.

11. Stay Hydrated:

- Hydrate before, during, and after
your somatic exercises.

- Water supports overall bodily
functions and aids in recovery.

12. Listen to Your Body:

   - Pay attention to how different foods make you feel.

   - Adjust your diet based on your individual needs and preferences.

Remember, these dietary suggestions are general guidelines, and individual needs may vary.

Chapter VIII.
Troubleshooting and
Common Mistakes

A. Addressing Discomfort

Addressing discomfort during somatic exercises is crucial to ensure a safe and effective practice. Here are mindful strategies to navigate and alleviate discomfort:

1. Gentle Exploration:

- Begin your somatic practice with gentle exploration.

- Gradually move into each exercise, paying close attention to sensations without pushing into discomfort.

2. Breath Awareness:

- Use your breath as a guide to manage discomfort.

- Inhale deeply to bring awareness to the area of discomfort, and exhale slowly, allowing tension to release.

3. Modification and Adaptation:

- Modify exercises to suit your comfort level.

- If a particular movement causes discomfort, adapt it or explore a gentler variation. The goal is to create a positive and nourishing experience for your body.

4. Mindful Movement:

- Emphasize mindful movement.

- Move slowly and with intention, avoiding abrupt or forceful actions. Mindful movement allows you to tune into your body's signals more effectively.

5. Progressive Approach:

- Progress gradually in intensity.

- If discomfort arises, consider stepping back to a more basic version of the exercise. Over time, you can slowly build up to more challenging movements.

6. Mind-Body Connection:

- Foster a strong mind-body connection.

- Cultivate awareness of the sensations in your body, distinguishing between discomfort and pain. Respond mindfully to ensure your practice remains positive and supportive.

7. Prop Support:

- Utilize props or support when needed.

- Props like cushions, blocks, or straps can provide assistance and help alleviate discomfort by modifying the range of motion or providing additional support.

8. Check Alignment:

- Assess your body's alignment during exercises.

- Misalignment may contribute to discomfort. Ensure proper posture and alignment, especially in weight-bearing activities.

9. Release and Relaxation:

- Include moments of intentional release and relaxation.

- After engaging in more active movements, take time for passive stretches or relaxation postures to release any accumulated tension.

10. Consultation with a Professional:

- If persistent discomfort or pain arises, consider consulting with a healthcare professional or a somatic instructor.

- They can provide personalized guidance, assess your movements, and offer tailored recommendations.

11. Mindful Endings:

- Conclude your somatic practice mindfully.

- Finish with gentle stretches or restorative postures to leave your body in a state of relaxation. This can contribute to an overall positive experience.

Remember that discomfort in somatic exercises should be addressed with care and attention. Listen to your body, honor its signals, and make adjustments as needed. A mindful and responsive approach to discomfort contributes to a sustainable and beneficial somatic practice over time. If in doubt or if discomfort persists, seeking guidance from a qualified somatic instructor or healthcare professional is advisable.

B. Adjusting Techniques for Individual Needs

Adjusting somatic techniques to individual needs is essential for a personalized and effective practice. Here are mindful strategies to tailor somatic exercises based on individual requirements:

1. Body Awareness Dialogue:

- Encourage a continuous dialogue with your body.

- Pay attention to the sensations, limitations, and comfort levels during each exercise. This awareness informs adjustments to cater to individual needs.

2. Customizing Intensity:

- Recognize that individuals have varying levels of flexibility and strength.

- Customize the intensity of movements to match the individual's current abilities. Gradually increase intensity as they become more comfortable with the exercises.

3. Prop Utilization:

- Incorporate props to enhance comfort and support.

- Props such as cushions, blocks, or straps can be used to modify movements and accommodate specific body needs. They provide additional support or modify the range of motion.

4. Range of Motion Adaptation:

- Adjust the range of motion based on individual capabilities.

- Modify movements to a range that feels comfortable for the individual. Gradually expand the range as their flexibility and comfort levels improve.

5. Individualized Breathing Techniques:

- Tailor breathing techniques to individual preferences.

- Some individuals may find certain breathing patterns more comfortable than others. Allow flexibility in breathing techniques to accommodate individual preferences.

6. Mindful Check-ins:

- Periodically check in with individuals during the practice.

- Ask for feedback on comfort, any areas of tension, or specific sensations. Adjust the exercises accordingly to ensure a positive and personalized experience.

7. Seated or Standing Options:

- Provide options for seated or standing variations.

- Some individuals may find seated postures more accessible, while others prefer standing. Offering variations allows individuals to choose what suits them best.

8. Mind-Body Connection Exploration:

- Encourage exploration of the mind-body connection.

- Individuals may have different levels of awareness regarding the mind-body connection. Guide them in exploring sensations and adapting movements based on their unique experiences.

9. Supportive Verbal Cues:

- Offer supportive verbal cues.

- Use positive and encouraging language to guide individuals through the movements. This helps build confidence and fosters a positive mindset during the practice.

10. Gradual Progression:

- Emphasize gradual progression.

- Tailor the pace of the somatic practice to align with the individual's comfort and readiness for advancement. Allow for a steady and supportive progression over time.

11. Individualized Modifications:

- Be open to modifying exercises based on specific needs.

- Individuals may have unique considerations such as injuries, chronic conditions, or physical limitations. Modify exercises to accommodate these individual factors.

12. Regular Check-ins and Adjustments:

- Regularly check in with individuals and be responsive to their needs.

- Somatic practices are dynamic, and needs may evolve over time. Regularly assess and adjust techniques to ensure ongoing comfort and alignment with individual requirements.

By embracing adaptability and mindful responsiveness, somatic exercises can be tailored to meet the diverse needs of individuals. This approach fosters a positive and inclusive somatic experience, promoting overall well-being and personal growth.

Chapter IX. Advanced Somatic Practices

A.   Building upon the Basics

Building upon the basics in somatic exercises involves progressing gradually, deepening your mind-body connection, and exploring more advanced movements. Here are steps to advance your somatic practice:

1. Mastery of Fundamentals:

- Ensure a solid foundation by mastering basic somatic exercises.

- Focus on refining your technique, awareness, and breath control in fundamental movements before progressing.

2. Gradual Intensity Increase:

- Introduce gradual increases in intensity.

- Explore variations of basic movements that challenge your range of motion, strength, and flexibility. Progress incrementally to avoid strain.

3. Mindful Breath Expansion:

- Deepen your breath awareness and control.

- Incorporate advanced breath practices such as extended inhalations, exhalations, or breath retention. Sync your breath with intricate movements for enhanced mindfulness.

4. Complex Movement Sequences:

- Combine multiple movements into complex sequences.

- Develop fluid transitions between different somatic exercises. This challenges your coordination and mind-body connection.

5. Targeted Muscle Engagement:

- Focus on specific muscle engagement.

- Isolate and activate individual muscles within a movement. This level of precision enhances muscle awareness and control.

6. Incorporate Flowing Transitions:

- Emphasize flowing transitions between exercises.

- Smooth, continuous movements improve the flow of your somatic practice. This builds grace and control in your body's responses.

7. Dynamic Stability Challenges:

- Introduce dynamic stability challenges.

- Engage in movements that require balance and stability, incorporating elements like one-legged stances or dynamic shifts to challenge your body's proprioception.

8. Exploration of Proprioception:

- Deepen your proprioceptive awareness.

- Practice somatic exercises blindfolded or with closed eyes to rely on your body's internal cues. This enhances sensory perception and mindfulness.

9. Somatic Meditation Practices:

- Include somatic meditation practices.

- Engage in longer periods of stillness, focusing on internal sensations. This promotes a deeper sense of embodiment and presence.

10. Creative Movement Exploration:

- Explore creative and intuitive movement.

- Allow spontaneous, free-form movements that arise naturally. This encourages self-expression and a deeper connection with your body.

11. Expert Guidance:

- Seek guidance from a somatic expert or advanced practitioner.

- Work with a qualified instructor to receive personalized feedback and guidance on refining advanced techniques.

12. Reflect and Adjust:

- Regularly reflect on your somatic practice.

- Assess your progress, note areas for improvement, and be open to adjusting your routine. A reflective approach supports ongoing growth.

As you build upon the basics, maintain a mindful and intuitive connection with your body. Listen to its signals, respect your limits, and enjoy the evolving journey of somatic exploration. Always prioritize safety and seek professional guidance if needed.

B. Fine-tuning Mind-Body Harmony

Fine-tuning mind-body harmony in somatic practices involves refining your awareness, deepening your connection, and cultivating a sense of balance. Here are mindful strategies for fine-tuning mind-body harmony:

1. Heightened Sensory Awareness:

- Cultivate heightened sensory awareness during movements.

- Pay attention to subtle changes in muscle tension, joint articulation, and breath. Sharpening your sensory perception deepens your mind-body connection.

2. Mindful Breath Integration:

- Integrate breath with heightened awareness.

- Explore nuanced breathing patterns, synchronizing breath

with specific movements. Use your breath as a guide to enhance presence and connection.

3. Progressive Relaxation Techniques:

- Incorporate progressive relaxation techniques.

- Systematically relax different muscle groups, progressing from head to toe. This promotes a profound sense of relaxation and awareness throughout the body.

4. Body-Scan Meditation:

- Practice body-scan meditation.

- Direct focused attention to each part of your body, observing sensations without judgment. This mindfulness practice enhances your ability to detect and release tension.

5. Slow and Controlled Movements:

- Emphasize slow and controlled movements.

- Execute somatic exercises with deliberate and intentional motions. This deliberate pace enhances precision and fosters a more profound mind-body connection.

6. Centering Techniques:

- Incorporate centering techniques.

- Explore methods such as grounding exercises or visualizations to center your awareness and promote a harmonious connection between mind and body.

7. Mindful Transitions:

- Pay attention to transitions between movements.

- Mindfully navigate the spaces between exercises, maintaining awareness even in moments of stillness. Transitions become opportunities for deepening your mind-body harmony.

8. Embodied Presence in Stillness:

- Cultivate embodied presence during stillness.

- When holding postures or in moments of rest, maintain a heightened awareness of your body. Allow stillness to become a rich experience of embodied presence.

9. Exploring Micro-Movements:

- Explore micro-movements within postures.

- Allow small, subtle movements to arise organically. This fine-tuning of micro-movements deepens your sensitivity to the intricacies of your body's responses.

10. Mindful Repetition:

- Engage in mindful repetition of movements.

- Revisit familiar somatic exercises with a focus on refining each repetition. This approach encourages a continuous process of refinement.

11. Intuitive Movement Practices:

- Incorporate intuitive movement practices.

- Allow your body to guide spontaneous movements, embracing a sense of freedom and creativity. This fosters a dynamic and intuitive mind-body connection.

12. Reflective Journaling:

- Maintain a reflective journal.

- Document your experiences, insights, and observations during somatic practices. This reflective process deepens your understanding and contributes to continuous refinement.

Fine-tuning mind-body harmony is an ongoing process that requires patience, curiosity, and a commitment to self-discovery. By incorporating these mindful strategies into your somatic practices, you can gradually enhance the subtleties of your

mind-body connection for a more
profound and harmonious
experience.

Chapter X. Frequently Asked Questions

A. Addressing Common Concerns

Here are 20 common questions often asked by individuals exploring somatic practices:

1. What exactly are somatic exercises?

- Somatic exercises involve mindful movement and breath awareness to improve physical and mental well-being.

2. How can somatic exercises benefit me?

- Benefits include improved flexibility, reduced tension, enhanced body awareness, and stress relief.

3. Can anyone practice somatic exercises?

   - Yes, somatic exercises are suitable for individuals of all fitness levels and ages.

4. Do I need any special equipment for somatic exercises?

   - Generally, no special equipment is required. Many exercises can be done with just a comfortable space.

5. How often should I practice somatic exercises?

   - Consistency is key. Starting with a few times per week and gradually increasing is recommended.

6. Are somatic exercises a form of meditation?

   - While there are meditative aspects, somatic exercises primarily focus on mindful movement and body awareness.

7. Can somatic exercises help with chronic pain?

- Yes, somatic exercises may assist in managing chronic pain by addressing muscular tension and improving movement patterns.

8. Is there a specific age range for somatic exercises?

- No, somatic exercises can be adapted for individuals of all ages, promoting lifelong well-being.

9. Can somatic exercises improve posture?

- Yes, somatic exercises often include movements to enhance posture and body alignment.

10. How long does it take to see results from somatic exercises?

- Results vary, but many people report feeling more relaxed and noticing changes in flexibility after a few weeks.

11. Are somatic exercises a form of yoga?

- While there are similarities, somatic exercises focus more on internal awareness and subtle movements than traditional yoga.

12. Can somatic exercises be done by people with injuries?

- It depends on the injury. Consult with a healthcare professional to determine suitable exercises for your condition.

13. Are there specific exercises for stress relief in somatics?

- Yes, many somatic exercises are designed to release tension and promote relaxation.

14. Can somatic exercises be done sitting or standing?

- Absolutely, somatic exercises can be adapted for various positions, including sitting and standing.

15. Is somatic education the same as somatic exercises?

- Somatic education may encompass a broader understanding of body-mind connection, while somatic exercises are specific movement practices.

16. Can somatic exercises help with anxiety?

- Yes, the focus on breath and body awareness in somatic exercises can be beneficial for managing anxiety.

17. How do somatic exercises differ from traditional fitness routines?

- Somatic exercises prioritize internal awareness, gentle movements, and releasing tension, distinguishing them from more vigorous workouts.

18. Are there specific exercises for improving sleep with somatics?

- Yes, certain somatic exercises may be beneficial for promoting relaxation and improving sleep quality.

19. Can I combine somatic exercises with other forms of exercise?

- Absolutely, somatic exercises can complement other activities and enhance overall well-being.

20. Are there risks associated with somatic exercises?

- Generally, somatic exercises are low risk. However, individuals with specific health concerns should consult with a healthcare professional before starting a new practice.

Chapter XI. Conclusion

A. Encouragement for Ongoing Practice

Embarking on a somatic journey is a commendable commitment to your well-being. As you continue your practice, here's some encouragement:

1. Celebrate Progress:

   - Acknowledge and celebrate even small achievements. Every step in your somatic journey is a valuable part of your progress.

2. Embrace Patience:

- Transformation takes time. Embrace patience and allow yourself the space to grow and evolve through your somatic practice.

3. Listen to Your Body:

- Your body is your guide. Listen to its signals, respect its limits, and be attuned to the wisdom it shares during your practice.

4. Embody Mindfulness:

- Infuse mindfulness into each movement. The more present you are, the deeper your mind-body connection will become.

5. Adapt and Modify:

   - Don't hesitate to adapt exercises to suit your needs. Your practice is uniquely yours, and modifications can enhance its effectiveness.

6. Consistency is Key:

   - Regularity amplifies the benefits of somatic exercises. Find a rhythm that works for you, and let your practice become a consistent part of your routine.

7. Reflect and Learn:

- Use reflective moments to learn about yourself. Journaling can be a powerful tool to track your progress, challenges, and insights.

8. Find Joy in Movement:

- Let joy be your companion in movement. When you find joy, your practice becomes a source of not only physical well-being but also genuine happiness.

9. Connect with Community:

- Consider joining or forming a somatic community. Sharing experiences and insights with others on a similar journey can be uplifting and inspiring.

10. Mind-Body Integration Off the Mat:

- Extend your somatic awareness beyond your practice sessions. Carry the principles of mindfulness and body connection into your daily life.

11. Be Kind to Yourself:

- Practice self-compassion. If some days feel challenging, acknowledge it with kindness, and know that each practice is an opportunity for growth.

12. Embrace the Journey:

   - Your somatic journey is an exploration, not a destination. Embrace the ongoing process of self-discovery and well-being.

Remember, your commitment to somatic exercises is an investment in your holistic health. With each breath and movement, you are nurturing a harmonious relationship between your mind and body. Keep going, stay curious, and enjoy the transformative journey ahead!

Conclusion

In conclusion, "Somatic Exercises for Beginners" invites you on a transformative journey towards enhanced well-being, mindfulness, and a harmonious mind-body connection. This book serves as a guide, providing a comprehensive exploration of somatic practices from the foundational basics to the fine-tuned nuances of advanced techniques.

As you delve into the world of somatic exercises, you've discovered the power of mindful movement, breath integration, and the profound impact it can have on your physical and mental health. From addressing common concerns to adjusting techniques for individual needs, you've embraced a personalized approach to your somatic practice.

The journey didn't stop at the basics but encouraged you to build upon them, introducing advanced concepts and fostering a deeper connection with your body. Through gentle encouragement, patience, and a commitment to progress, you've fine-tuned the harmony between your mind and body.

The book emphasizes the joy found in movement, the significance of listening to your body, and the art of adapting exercises to suit your unique needs. Whether you're a beginner or an advanced practitioner, the principles outlined in this book provide a foundation for a lifelong somatic practice.

As you continue this journey, remember to celebrate each step, practice self-compassion, and find joy in the ongoing process of self-discovery. Your commitment to somatic exercises is a testament to your dedication to holistic well-being, and the benefits will extend far beyond the pages of this book.

May your somatic practice be a source of inspiration, growth, and mindful living. Here's to a harmonious and flourishing journey ahead!